FORGET THE DIET:

10 KEY HABITS FOR LIVING A HOLISTIC LIFESTYLE FROM THE INSIDE OUT

By

Cathyann Greenidge, CHHC
Certified Holistic Health Counselor

CONTENT

SPIRIT

SOUL

BODY

Forget the Diet: 10 Key Habits

Forget the Diet: 10 Key Habits

Acknowledgement

I want to acknowledge my mom, who 'til this day believes that I have the answer to every question that she asks me. Sometimes I do and other times some research is necessary. I always remember when I was 11 years old and was about to start secondary school (high school) in the Caribbean and someone in the neighborhood had made a negative comment about whether I deserved to be attending such a top rank secondary school. My mom defended me and I always remembered that. She instilled in me that I could do anything I set my mind to. I thank God for her and would not change the way I was raised for anything because it taught me independence, street smarts and confidence.

I also want to acknowledge you for taking the time to read this life enhancing source and I pray that it will be a blessing to you and whomever you share the information with.

NB: The information in this book is for educational purposes and is not intended to replace the advice of your doctor or any medical professional whose care you are under. Always consult your doctor / medical practitioner whenever you plan to make a significant change to your diet / health routine.

Introduction

Spirit, Soul & Body

We are spirit beings with a soul (place of our mind, will, emotions & intellect) and we live in a body.

In the process of writing this book my goal was to make it simple. I wanted those of you who are ripe and ready to make effective and positive changes to your health to be able to have something to get you started and to use as a reference.

In life we acquire habits whether they are beneficial to our well being or not. According to the Random House College Dictionary, a habit is an acquired behavior pattern regularly followed until it has become almost involuntary. So keep that in mind as you read this book.

Forget the Diet: 10 Key Habits

The ten key habits that I write about are some of the foundational things that have been and continue to be important for me as I implement good health habits. We are spirit beings, we have a soul and we live in a body. Many people in our communities do not acknowledge that God created this earth and everything in it but the Bible makes it clear that, "the earth is the Lord's, and everything in it."

It is very difficult for me to look at this world and the order that exists and not believe that God took his time and planned out the foundational consistent things just so. In Genesis, it states that God created the earth in six days and rested on the seventh. When you read this just remember that we are finite and governed by time, God is not since he is infinite, knowing the beginning and the end. Our day is limited to 24 hours, his has no limit.

Forget the Diet: 10 Key Habits

We have four seasons here in America and in the Caribbean where I am from we have two seasons, the dry season and the rainy season. Things like that do not happen by chance. There has to be an almighty powerful creator to pull off something like that. This is why we can plan our vacations based on the seasons and be able to know that in the summer it is hot and in winter it is cold.

Wouldn't you think that it was crazy if from one year to the next, you were not sure if summer would be hot or winter would be cold? That would be crazy and we would not be able to rely on the seasons to plan our activities. That would sure confuse the farmers and we would not be able to have consistent plant food.

Isn't it a relief to know that in the Bible, God told Noah that as long as this earth remains there will be seed time and harvest time and seasons, and to top it off he gave us a divine promise that he would not flood the entire earth again. He demonstrates this through the rainbow so whenever I see a rainbow, I remember this promise and I thank God for his word that never fails.

I love that I can rely on the God who created this earth and gave us bodies to be able to function on this earth according to His divine order of things. This leads me to the following bible verse

Mark 2:17 NLT

"…healthy people don't need a doctor - sick people do… "

This verse reminds me that I have a purpose which is to help those who seek me out to help them Create, Live and Love their Holistic

Forget the Diet: 10 Key Habits

Lifestyle. Also, when you really think about it, in our society we usually go to the doctor only when something is wrong. We tend to focus on maintaining our health only after there has been an interruption in our wellbeing. Otherwise we go through our days eating what we want and doing what we want either because that is what we were taught --- it makes us happy or it satisfies an immediate need.

Well, one of my major goals is to assist individuals, like yourself, to take a preventative and maintenance approach to your health. My goal is not to turn you into a so called perfect healthy person because only God can provide perfection.

My goal is to empower you to make the best healthy choices based on your traditions, culture, personal preferences and economics

Forget the Diet: 10 Key Habits

and trust me, I know that everyone will not decide to become a vegetarian or only eat raw foods. There are those of you who will continue to eat meat, then obtaining the best quality meat should be your ultimate goal.

As I continue to improve my Holistic Lifestyle I am constantly reminded of a regular comment by Dr. A. R. Bernard to keep everything in balance and not do anything in extreme because it will only lead to error. So let me offer you a sneak peek into my process and believe me, I have not arrived. I still have work to do.

I Pray That This Will Be a Blessing To You ☺

Spirit

When your spirit is

in relationship

with God, you are

HOLY

Key Habit #1
Creating and Maintaining a Spiritual Connection with God

He is the creator of everything. He is the reason we exist so we should always honor and thank Him for all that he has done for us and all that we will do. So if you truly understand your purpose in this life and have had a glimpse of your future, you will thank him even when things may look horrible in the natural. You do this because you know deep in your spirit, that better days are coming and things will not always be like this.

I continually seek to grow and mature in my spiritual walk by praying and meditating because this is what sustains me when I feel like it is not worth it to be healthy and it would have been easier to just eat that piece of fried chicken. However, since I know my purpose on this earth, I just have to trust God to lead the way and order my steps as I make necessary plans. When I really think about it, it is really not about me, but about those I am here to help. A very wise person once told me that I should not ask, "Why am I here?" but instead, ask, "Who am I here for?"

Soul

When your soul is

in relationship with

God, you are

HAPPY

Key Habit #2
Perfecting Your Purpose on This Earth

Each one of us has been created for a purpose whether we know it or accept it. In 2005, as I started to take control of my health, I went through a soul searching process to help me find out my true purpose in life. I just had this heaviness in my soul with a deep need help my community in a positive way according the plan God had for my life.

In 2005, I read "The Purpose Driven Life: What on Earth Am I Here For?" by Rick Warren, to help me with the process of finding my purpose. I was so excited to find out what my purpose was, that, I read it once on my own and then again with a friend. Reading it the second time was very inspirational because Lisa and I would meet on the phone at night after consuming our daily reading. These

Forget the Diet: 10 Key Habits

opportunities, helped to develop my praise and worship skills as well as my ability to pray proficiently.

After we completed our sessions, I was lead into a forty day fast. During the fast I read "Perfecting Your Purpose: 40 Days to a More Meaningful Life" by David Ireland. Also, during this, time I did not consume any chicken, beef, pork or lamb. The only animal protein I ate was fish which was consume in the last 5 days of my fast. I made it through but it was interesting to feel the effects of the different categories of foods on my body.

In the first week, I ate only raw foods - fruits, vegetables and nuts (usually a salad combined from these groups without dressing – adding fruits and vegetables like apple, pineapple, craisins, avocado, cucumbers, pickles, olives and tomatoes made it easier to eat the mueslin greens). The next week, I added carbohydrates (breads) and subsequently, cooked foods (rice, grains and sweet-potato). In the final week, I added fish.

When I was just eating raw foods, I had energy like you would not believe. I was up each morning before my alarm clock. I felt really good. It was like I was floating. As I added carbohydrates and cooked foods, I started to feel more grounded and focused. However, if I had too much I became somewhat sluggish.

From what my body went through, I consequently would adjust my food intake to facilitate the energy level I needed for my day of planned activities. It was great when I had time to do it but if I had a hectic day and would eat what was available, I could not wait for my next opportunity to get back on track. It is wonderful when you have that control

Forget the Diet: 10 Key Habits

over your own body and you choose what will fuel it. Food is then used for its main purpose as fuel and not to soothe an emotional issue. Please note that I did not get to this stage in my live over night, it was, and still is, a journey.

After my period of fasting, I had clarity on my purpose and started the steps to walk it out.

Forget the Diet: 10 Key Habits

Key Habit #3
Involvement in Honest and Healthy Relationships

When embarking on a relationship you must always look at what you are bringing to this relationship, not just what the other person is bringing. It all starts with you because you are the only person you have power to control. Trying to manipulate and control is a form of witchcraft and you do not want to go there. Below are some exerpts from "Breaking UnGodly Soul Ties" by Michael Pitts. The goal is to get you thinking and focused on your current relationships and how you can make them better.

SELF-AUTHORITY – produces reliability. Your emotional well-being is not in the hands of others. No one can make you be what you don't want to be. The expectations of another do not determine how you will react to life's events.   No one can make you mad because you are in charge of your soul.   No one can drive you crazy because you've taken the keys out of their hands. If you are not in charge of yourself, any little thing can set you off. However, if you are in control of your soul, a temporary problem will not cause you to react in a drastic manner.

God will not place His approval on a relationship if helping them is hurting you. The relationship that is in a godly covenant gives and receives with joy. ...we are servants to all ... we should be slaves to none.   A godly relationship does not manipulate through anger, but motivates through love.   When a sound comes from a merry heart, it comes in the form of laughter.

With regards to my relationships, I have always taken time out to meditate on my relations with others and how I can make them stronger and better. I am purposeful with my relationships.   I do not create "willy-nilly" relationships so the ones that I allow myself to be part of receive genuine time from me. I also focus on the following teachings which emphasizes that relationships have 4 stages – introduction, acquaintance, friendship and intimacy.

People therefore fall into either one of these categories so be very careful not to allow someone to enter a level of relationship with you that they are not prepared for. It will become strained when you have to reposition them. If this is you and you have to reposition someone, please let the Holy Spirit lead you and not do it in your own strength as this is a difficult task with a tendency for feelings to be hurt.

Key Habit #4
Create & Nourish a Strong Purposeful Support System by Eating with Others Whenever Possible

When I eat with others, my focus is not on the food - it is on the person who chose to spend time with me. As we converse, my fork/spoon is on the plate between bites. This significantly decreases my chances of overeating. Research shows that it takes our brain approximately 20 minutes to register that we are full. So when I take my time and chew each bite completely while enjoying my company, I allow the digestive enzymes do their job.

Spending Quality Time with Those Who Inspire Me

We all need to be encouraged and nurtured. It is known that babies that are not cuddled and nurtured have a delay in their development

Forget the Diet: 10 Key Habits

and this principle applies to anything that is newly birthed. Whether it is a new level in life or a new job, you need to be supported by others who have been there before or others who know someone who has been there before and can relate in some positive and helpful way.

I am very careful who I let speak into my life and even when someone does, I am always checking to make sure it lines up with God's word. Also when my emotional needs are met through counseling with those more mature than I, there is a significant decrease in the need to be emotionally fed by food. So I thank God for all the strong teachings that I have received from those who are more spiritually mature than I.

Body

When your body is

in relationship with

God, you are

HEALTHY

The body needs to rest in order to heal and if you do not take time out to rest, it will make you rest by becoming sick or shutting down to protect itself. One of the focus areas in Holistic Health Counseling is primary foods and these include spirituality, relationships, career, and physical activity. In focusing on having time to revive myself, I devote time to God in the morning upon waking and in the evening before I go to sleep. Something else, I practice, is constant communication with Him throughout the day.

Key Habit #5
Cleansing the Colon

I had my first colonic in the fall of 2006. At the time, I was hosting a radio show called "Conscious Health" which aired in Bronx, NY. My co-host Deanna, a Colon Therapist and a Massage Therapist, provided me with my first colonic. I decided to get it done primarily for my health and also to be able to speak from a place of experience when I recommended it to clients.

Subsequently, I became a Colon Therapist and for the next 2 year I graduated from having one every three months with the seasons to 1-4 a month depending on what going on with my body. I have since added herbs to my daily routine and with continued implementation of healthier choices I have decreased my need for frequent sessions. Also related to colon health, there is something that I have added to my daily routine that I cannot function without and that is my step stool. I put it in front of my toilet and place my feet on it during a bowel movement. I learned from my colon therapist and then in Colon Hygiene School, that squatting is the correct position for complete elimination of waste from our bodies, not sitting like we are at the dining table having a meal.

This was a powerful revelation for me. Now I pass it on to you to help you with your Holistic Lifestyle process. Share it with your friends and family because they need to know. There are so many simple things we can implement to stay healthy. We just need to filter through the fluff and get to the core foundational information. Simplicity is much less stressful than complicated multistep processes. I don't need all the extra stuff. Just get to the point.

Forget the Diet: 10 Key Habits

On 1/26/08, at the Christian Cultural Center Single's Launch Meeting, Chris Burge stated that experience is the slow way that God teaches us and revelation is the fastest. I don't know about you, but if I can learn and understand something that is helpful to me quickly and clearly instead of multistep and drawn out, I always choose the former.

Forget the Diet: 10 Key Habits

Key Habit #6
Detoxing the Body

I periodically drink Young Living's Balance Complete shake and Dr. Schulze's Superfood Plus as meal replacements. They are very filling – I always add some frozen or fresh fruit to the blender. I also use Juvaflex and Juva Cleanse essential oil blends internally (one drop on my tongue or in a 4oz of water). Rubbing one drop over my liver – the largest gland in the body with the primary function of cleansing and detoxifying the body – is very effective as well. I use these oils periodically and also every time I get a colonic. To learn how to get creative with making a Balance Complete Shake, go to the "My Holistic Recipes" section at the end of this book. Living this Holistic Lifestyle is all about techniques – putting things in place to help you succeed easily and with minimal stress.

Key Habit #7
Pay Attention to your DIET – add
therapeutic grade essential oils /
digestive enzymes / probiotics /
healthy fats

DIET

DIET is an interesting word because it has become that word that when people say it, they automatically think of some program that requires them to take part in some form of daily ritual that requires lots and lots of will power and if they do not maintain this ritual that was created by someone else, they fail.

Well, I am here to tell you that the way we eat, is, our diet whether it is healthy or unhealthy. It is not this step by step system that someone created to get their piece of the wellness market pie. It is listening to our bodies and eating according to our daily energy

Forget the Diet: 10 Key Habits

requirements for completing our activities.

I tell you this, when you start taking action to create your own Holistic Lifestyle, you will be amazed at how your body speaks to you. It is very intelligent. Just give it a chance to teach you a thing or two about yourself. You will be glad you did.

The dictionary defines diet as – food habitually provided. I chose this definition, because, it gives us education as well as shows that the food that is habitually provided can be whatever we choose it to be. Now, you know that I am going to encourage you to habitually provide your body with healthy food and remember baby steps so you do not sabotage your process and abort it early. You need to go through the growing incubation process and bring this new approach to your health to full term so that you can give birth.

Forget the Diet: 10 Key Habits

After you give birth to it, you now have to keep nurturing it and eventually, you will automatically chose foods that are good for your body and not tarry with the baby stuff. It needs more nurturing in the beginning like a new born baby but as it develops, it begins to take care of itself and you will begin to say things like, "I wish I had done this earlier. I wasted so much time. This is easier than I thought."

Therapeutic Grade Essential Oils / Digestive Enzymes / Probiotics

Now, let's refocus on the topic at hand. During my studies at the Institute for Integrative Nutrition (IIN) where I obtained my Certification, as a Holistic Health Counselor, I received a wealth of information on nutrition. One of the topics, was, the use of digestive enzymes and probiotics to assist with

Forget the Diet: 10 Key Habits

the digestion of food. I understood it but I really did not get into it until I learned about Young Living Essential Oils and their oil based supplements.

Young Living Essential Oils carry a line of digestive enzymes that can help you to digest just about any food you put in your mouth, chew and swallow. It was a very exciting time for me when I was introduced to these products because after I completed my studies at IIN, I started thinking about what I could offer my future clients in addition to health counseling. My focus immediately turned to oils and four months later, God connected Linda and I.

This was a wonderful start to my career as a health practitioner. Now I have a wonderful arsenal to choose from. Some of my personal favorites are Peppermint essential oil, Di-gize

Forget the Diet: 10 Key Habits

essential oil blend and Detoxzymes digestive enzymes as I use them regularly to help me digest cooked foods. To learn more about these products or to purchase you can go to the resource section of this book.

Probiotics

Probiotics are live microbial organisms that are naturally present in the digestive tract and vagina.

Probiotics are considered beneficial and are sometimes referred to as "friendly" bacteria. Some of the ways they are thought to promote health include suppressing the growth of potentially harmful bacteria, improving immune function, enhancing the protective barrier of the digestive tract, and helping to produce vitamin K (very important in clotting of blood to promote healing.

Forget the Diet: 10 Key Habits

There are over 400 species of microorganisms in the human digestive tract, including Lactobacillus and Bifidobacterium. A number of medical, diet, and lifestyle factors are believed to disturb the balance in the colon. This imbalance is called dysbiosis. Factors include:

- Inadequate dietary fiber
- Oral antibiotic therapy
- Infant formula feeding
- Ingestion of environmental toxins

Probiotics can be found in cultured dairy products such as yogurt or kefir, however, the number of live organisms varies greatly from product to product due to differences in processing methods. Fermented foods such as sauerkraut also contain probiotics.

Forget the Diet: 10 Key Habits

Healthy Fats

It should be shocking but I am not at all shocked at how we have been so brain washed through print ads and radio/TV commercial media to believe that the natural fats God provided for us like those in coconut, flax seed and avocado are bad but the imitation margarines and artificial butter products are better. Because it says low fat or heart healthy on the container does not mean that it is healthier!!!! Pleeeeeeze wake up and start asking questions to yourself and the manufacturers. They all have contact information on their packages. God's creations are always the correct version as long as they have not been tampered with by man.

When man starts meddling, we do not know what to expect. Wake up people. Nothing imitation can be as good as the original. We

Forget the Diet: 10 Key Habits

will buy original, name brand clothes, bags and shoes (the outer things) but we will skimp on what we put in our bodies (the inner things). What shows up on the outside is a reflection of what has been going on inside but you may have heard it this way before, "what happens in the dark will soon come to light."

If our bodies are not in a working, healthy state, how can we then enjoy these original, name brand things anyway? We need to check our priorities. What are we spending our money and time on? Does it help someone in a positive way? Think, think, think, think --- who are you here for?

Start taking back your health from the grips of major corporations who care more about making money than your health!!!!!!!!!!!!!!!! The same people, who sell you unhealthy products, take your money, fund sports arenas and their

Forget the Diet: 10 Key Habits

executives are hanging out in spas eating very healthy and being pampered. Don't you think you deserve to eat healthy and be pampered also?

Forget the Diet: 10 Key Habits

Key Habit #8
Chewing Food & Drinking Water

Chewing

"Throw it down your neck and taste it later." Horrifying thought isn't it but that is what many of us do now or used to do. We are in such a hurry these days that we do not take the time to chew and taste our foods. I heard the story of a gentleman, very busy business executive, who would eat fast food for breakfast, lunch and dinner in his car because he needed to make the best use of his time for meeting with clients.

Anyway, he was always in a hurry and rushed his food. He started working with a health counselor and one of the recommendations was to carve out time to actually sit and chew his food because even though he was seeking

Forget the Diet: 10 Key Habits

health counseling, he was not willing to give up his fast food. Well, lo and behold, as he started to actually chew and taste his food, he realized that he really did not like those burgers anyway.

This opened the door for his counselor to recommend some healthy alternatives. Isn't it amazing what your body will reveal to you once you use your parts the way God intended instead of abusing them. The teeth were made to chew so use them to chew. The stomach was make to mix and help digest your food, please do not make it chew by swallowing chunks of food by chewing 3 – 5 times before swallowing.

You should chew until you food is liquid especially carbohydrates since they are mainly digested in the mouth by amylase in your saliva. Oh, by the way, the phrase that I used

Forget the Diet: 10 Key Habits

earlier to start this topic was a phrase used by my Drill Sergeant in Army Basic Training. Never thought about what that did to my body but now I understand and because I know better, I do better. Now it is your turn to chew your food.

Drinking Water

I also increased my water intake. This did not happen overnight. I used to be a juice, Coco Rico (coconut soda) and Sprite drinker. Water was an occasional thing. The winter of 2002, was the beginning of my reunion with the love of drinking water. This occurred after completing my first colon cleanse, which lasted 2 weeks.

The protocol for this cleanse required that I take capsules and drink this powder that I

Forget the Diet: 10 Key Habits

mixed with natural apple juice – I did not make time to juice so I just bought it at the supermarket. I was allowed to eat salads and fruits only if I needed to and I was required to drink at least 8 glasses of water a day.

It was a very interesting time. Two days before I was to complete this cleanse, I wanted to quit. I felt like I had had enough but I persevered and completed it. I lost 7 pounds and felt really good. I then wanted to juice everything and cleanse every three months.

I, however, did not juice everything or cleanse every three months but this really put me back on track with my health since the previous 2 years weren't some of my best eating habit years. I was in graduate school then and assignments, working and getting as much sleep as I could in between took priority over what I ate. I just ate what was available and it did not help that there was a snack table set up in the back of the classroom.

Classes were all day the weekends I attended so I would snack all day to stay awake, and to some degree, out of boredom. I just kept packing on the pounds. This was the first time in my life I weighed over 200 pounds – I did not like it at all, but my health had been put on the back burner because I could not afford to fail graduate school. I was laser focused about completing my degree.

Well, after that cleanse, I started paying more attention to what I ate. When I shopped for groceries, I would only buy apple juice, orange juice and lots of fruits and vegetables. When I drank juice, I diluted it with water, because, after the colon cleanse, my sweet taste buds were more sensitive. Anything with added sugar just tasted too sweet. Slowly but surely my water intake increased to the point now that I will go months drinking mainly water and periodically tea or fresh juice from the juicer. Now I crave water to the point that if I forget my water bottle at home and have to drink water from a cup, I anticipate getting home to fill my 32 oz stainless steel bottle with water so I can drink as I need it.

I now juice fruits and vegetables periodically and prepare most of my meals at home. I also found out about Trader Joes in 2003, which was a God-send because now I do not have to go to a regular super market and be distracted by all these companies trying to take money out my pocket for nutrient deficient foods. Trader Joe's carry their own brand and the prices are cheaper. I love it but even there I have to read labels. I also shop at Whole Foods Market so that I can obtain as much organic items as my budget will handle.

Key Habit #9
Move Your Body

I am not an expert when it comes to exercising so I recommend that you seek out someone who is. However I do know and understand the benefits of exercise and some form of physical activity. When it comes to physical activity, I am not one for going to a gym but get me involved in a physical sport activity like volleyball and I am good. I also love to walk in nature. Not able to do much of that in New York City, but I love it just the same. Maybe I should move further away from NYC. Hmmmmm, that's a thought.

Balance

When all the parts (Spirit, Soul & Body) are functioning totally in harmony with GOD, there is righteousness, peace and joy.

Key Habit #10
Keep It All in Balance

In getting my health on track so that I could help others effectively, I am now trained as a Certified Holistic Health Counselor and a Certified Colon Hygienist. My main goal is to help those who seek my assistance in obtaining a healthy life. This is my purpose and the plan I believe God has for my life. Bill Hybels puts it this way, "what is your Holy discontent? That thing that when it bubbles up inside of you and you become like Popeye and you start to say, that's all I can stand and I can't stands no more."

Well, I cannot stand that people will sit and let a commercial, paid for by a corporation, dictate what they eat. Many of us are dealing with lifestyle diseases that could have been avoided.

Forget the Diet: 10 Key Habits

My maternal grandmother for instance had diabetes and dealt with all of its complications while taking a pharmacy of medications every day. My paternal grandmother had both of her legs amputated before she passed on due to the complications of her diabetes.

Even though it is present on both sides of my family, I choose not to be a victim of such an ailment. I will continually make wise choices when it comes to my diet. I will not do anything in extreme because as Dr. A. R. Bernard teaches, that only leads to error. I also do my best to pay attention to my food combinations when I am at home. At other people's homes I have no control so I always carry Di-Gize and Peppermint oils from, Young Living Essential Oils, in my oil bag to help with my food digestion.

Forget the Diet: 10 Key Habits

I am also constantly studying to expand my knowledge base in order to continue to be a blessing to those who are seeking to change their health situation.

With regards to career, I created a work schedule to facilitate alone time but even though I created it that way I still have to fight off those things that come in my way to steal my time. It is a battle but the structure is in place; I just have to continually use it and so do you.

Now I implore you to look at these "10 Key Habits" and decide within yourself, which one is the easiest for you to implement. Then all you need to do is be consistent for 3 weeks (21 day) and voila, you have created a healthy habit. Do it. It's fun. Your body will like it.

<u>Appendix A</u>
<u>Resources</u>

Forget the Diet: 10 Key Habits

Bibliography

Essential Oils Desk Reference Edited by Essential Science Publishing

African Holistic Health by Dr. Llaila O. Afrika

Rawsome Recipes by Robin Boyd

Raw Food Bible by Craig B. Sommers

Merck Manual of Medicine Information, 2nd Home Edition, Published April 2003

Breaking Ungodly Soul Ties by Michael Pitts, M.A.P.S Institute, Swanson, OH, 1997

Caldwell, Bettye. May, 1998. "Early experiences shape social development." *Child Care Information Exchange*: 53-59.

Isabella, Russell A. 1993. "Origins of attachment: Maternal interactive behavior across the first year." *Child Development*, 64: 605-621.

Forget the Diet: 10 Key Habits

PRODUCTS

To purchase quality organic unadulterated essential oils, oil based supplements and skin care products: www.youngliving.us or call (800) 371-3515 and use member referral # 918570

Step Stool: I purchased mine from Walmart in the hardware department. It was $9.99

Appendix B
Healthy Kitchen Additions

Forget the Diet: 10 Key Habits

Cooking Equipment
> Stainless steel pots/pans
> Wooden spoons/spatulas

Spices
> Seas salt

Natural Sweetener
> Agave

Whole Grains
> Quinoa
> Bulgar Wheat Berries
> Amaranth

Good Fats
> Flaxseeds (add to shakes/cereals)
> Avocado (add to shakes/salads)
> Coconut Oil (use to cook)
> Unsalted butter (no margarine)
> Olive oil for salads (use cold)

Good Proteins
> Nuts
> Beans

Calcium
> Greens (Kale, Collard)

Appendix C
Recipes

Forget the Diet: 10 Key Habits

Some of My Holistic Lifestyle Recipes & Tips

When I prepare these recipes, I use primarily organic items but I know that everyone's budget is not the same so use what you have and enjoy☺ ☺

Equipment You May Need To Be Successful With These Recipes

High Powered Blender (I use the Vitamix)

Food Processor

Products You Will Need To Be Successful With These Recipes

Balance Complete

Organic Therapeutic Grade Essential Oils and Oil Blends

(In order to obtain the above products you will need to create a wholesale account with Young Living Essential Oils. To get started you can go to www.youngliving.us or call

(800)371-3515 and use the member referral # 918570

Balance Complete Shake

Makes 2 Thick Servings (~ 8 oz each)

Ingredients:

12 oz of milk (almond or rice) – use water if you prefer

2 scoops of Balance Complete Powder

½ cup of frozen fruit (berries & peaches are my favorites)

1 table spoon of flax meal

Method:

Pour milk into blender

Add two scoops of Balance Complete

Blend until completely mixed (I start on low and increase speed)

Add frozen fruit and blend until completely mixed

Add flax meal and blend until completely mixed

Pour into glass and enjoy with a straw or pour into your favorite polycarbonate bottle and drink throughout the day (I do either one depending on whether I am home or going to work)

Forget the Diet: 10 Key Habits

Dairy Free Hot Cereal

Makes approximately 4 servings
2 step process because soaking ingredients overnight is required

Ingredients:
5 cups of boiled water
1 cup of steel cut oats
½ cup of raw cashews
½ cup of raw almonds
2 tablespoons of raw pumpkin seeds
2 tablespoons of dried cranberries
2 tablespoons of dried wolfberries (gogi berries)
2 tablespoons of flax meal

Method:
Boil 3 cups of water
Place all ingredients except flax meal in a stainless steel mixing bowl/glass mixing bowl or medium size casserole dish

Pour water over ingredients and let soak overnight

In the morning boil 2 cups of water and pour into blender

Add all ingredients and blend

Then place all blended ingredients into an appropriate size saucepan and gently heat on lowest setting stirring continuously until desired temperature – do not boil

Stir in flax meal

Pour desired amount into bowl sit and enjoy – Don't forget to chew

You may not need to sweeten due to predigested carbohydrates and dried fruit

Apple Wolfberry (Gogi Berry) Pie

(Adapted from Raw Foods Bible by Craig B. Sommers – Almost Famous Apple Pie)

Makes 1 deep dish pie or 2 shallow dish pies – 8 servings

Crust Ingredients:

2 cups of raw almonds (soaked 12-24 hours)

2 cups of pitted dates

4 drops of orange or lemon from Young Living   Essential Oils

Filling Ingredients:

9-12 organic apples (I use gala or fuji)

1 cup of dried wolfberries (gogi berries) – soaked several hours in just enough water to cover them

2 tablespoons of flax meal/slippery elm or psyllium powder (I use the flax meal)

2 teaspoons of cinnamon powder
¼ teaspoon of nutmeg powder

To Make Crust:
Place all crust ingredients in a food processor and process with the S blade until it resembles dough. Press into pie dish (I use a glass pie dish).

To Make Filling:
Core and chop the apples into medium size pieces. Place half the apples into food processor along with the rest of the ingredients, including the water from the soaking wolfberries, and process until smooth. Set aside the mixture in a mixing bowl. Place the rest of the apples in the food processor and pulse until a chunky texture is achieved. Mix the batches together. Pour into the pie shell

and enjoy!!!!!!!!!!!!!! Place in the refrigerator for a few hours to allow the filling to become firm.

Forget the Diet: 10 Key Habits

No Mayonnaise Tuna Salad

(Adapted from Rosanda Richardson's Personal Recipe)

Enough to make 2 -3 sandwiches

Ingredients:

1 6oz can of tuna

Juice of 1 lemon or lime

1 tablespoon of dried cranberries

Sea salt to taste

Pepper sauce to taste (this is a Caribbean condiment but you can spice up your tuna however you choose)

Method

Open can of tuna and empty contents into a small bowl

Cut lemon/lime in half, remove seeds and squeeze onto tuna

Cut cranberries into tiny pieces and add to bowl

Add sea salt to taste

Add pepper sauce to taste

Use a fork to mash and mix ingredients

There you have it now you can serve it however you choose

I usually make a sandwich with sprout cinnamon raisin bread so that I can have my sweet/salt combination. That way I do not crave anything else after I am finished.

You can have it on your choice of whole grain crackers as well.

(*This will tap into just about every taste bud in your mouth*)

Forget the Diet: 10 Key Habits

Cold/Flu Relief Tea

Makes 1 Serving – This recipe uses only Young Living Essential Oils Therapeutic Grade Essential Oils and that is what I recommend if you are going to try this recipe. I know that these oils are pure and I therefore cannot vouch for another company's oils.

Ingredients:
1 cup (8 oz) of water
2 teaspoon of agave to sweeten
2 drops of Thieves oil
4 drops of citrus oil of your choice (Lemon/Tangerine/Orange/Grapefruit)
1 drop of Peppermint (WARNING: 1 drop is enough - equal to 28 cups of peppermint tea made from tea bags. So inhale the vapors from the rim of the cup. Do not put your face over the cup)

Method:

Boil water

Drop oils into teacup

Add agave to sweeten, if desired

Pour water into cup stir and enjoy!!!!!!!!!!!!!!!!!!!!!!

(Make this tea and drink as often as you need or every 2-4 hours if you want to get well again naturally. I make it whenever I feel something trying to take over my system – sore throat, ear ache or stuffy nose. It knocks it out)

Forget the Diet: 10 Key Habits

About The Author

Cathyann Greenidge immigrated to the United States from Barbados in 1990. At a young age, she was always concerned about the health and well-being of others and knew she wanted to be a Dietician. That, however, did not materialize because she joined the US Army Reserves 6 months after entering this country and was given the Military Occupational Specialty (MOS) of Occupational Therapy (OT) Specialist. This is a field that she fell in love with and is still part of now more than 17 years later as she currently holds a Masters Degree.

Forget the Diet: 10 Key Habits

During her 8 years of military service, she did in fact also become a Licensed Practical Nurse, graduating in June 1998. Still not feeling like she was truly walking in her purpose she sought God on this matter and in 2005 she embarked on her journey of becoming a Holistic Practitioner so she could help people to regain and/or maintain their health with minimal use of processed and preservative ridden foods.

In continuing to be obedient to God and walk in her purpose, she then furthered her education by becoming a Certified Holistic Health Counselor and a Certified Colon Hygienist. She realizes that every person she works with is

Forget the Diet: 10 Key Habits

different so she needs an arsenal of modalities so she can help everyone who seeks her assistance even if it is just to provide a referral to a specialist like a Chiropractor.

To Contact Author:
cathyann@myholisticlifestyle.com